Essential Home Remedies

STAYING HEALTHY WITH SIMPLE, NATURAL HOME REMEDIES FROM THE PANTRY AND THE GARDEN

SUE WOLEDGE

Copyright © 2012 by Sue Woledge

All rights reserved.

No portion of this book may be reproduced in any form without written permission from the publisher or author.

DISCLAIMER: THIS PUBLICATION IS *designed to share the Author's opinion and understanding regarding the subject matter covered. Whilst every effort is made to ensure that the information herein is correct, the Author specifically disclaims any personal liability, loss or risk incurred because of the use, misuse and application either directly or indirectly of any advice or information herein. Any reliance you place on such information is therefore strictly at your own risk.*

Contents

Dedication	1
1. How It All Started	4
2. The Digestive Healer: Slippery Elm	11
What Is Slippery Elm?	
How To Take Slippery Elm	
How Do I Use Slippery Elm?	
3. A Natural Antibiotic: Garlic	20
How Do I Use Garlic?	
4. Lose Weight & Lower Blood Pressure With Chili	27
How Do I Use Chili?	

5. The Healer: Aloe Vera 32
   Make Your Own Aloe Vera Juice
   How Do I Use Aloe Vera?

6. From Cancer to Morning Sickness: Ginger 37
   How Do I Use Ginger?

7. Thyme For Coughs and Colds 41
   Use Thyme For Coughs
   How Do I Use Thyme?

8. The Master Alkaliser: Lemon 48
   How Do I Use Lemon?

9. From Breast Milk to Farts: Fennel Seed 52
   How Do I Use Fennel?

10. Breath Deep and Be Calm with Lemon Balm 56
    How Do I Use Lemon Balm?

11. The Swiss Army Knife: Lavender Essential Oil 60
    How Do I Use Lavender Essential Oil?

12. Breathe Easy with Peppermint Essential Oil 64
    How Do I Use Peppermint Oil?

13. Used For Almost Everything: Apple Cider 67
    Vinegar
       How Do I Use Apple Cider Vinegar?

14. From Gout To Cleaning: Baking Soda 71
       Baking Soda as A Cancer Treatment
       Baking Soda for Odors Including Bad Breath
       How To Take Baking Soda

15. More Handy Remedies 77
       Activated Charcoal
       Bach Rescue Remedy
       Coriander
       Honey
       Juicing

16. Recipes & Reminders 89
       Slippery Elm
       Garlic
       Chili
       Aloe Vera
       Ginger
       Thyme
       Lemon
       Fennel

    Lemon Balm
    Apple Cider Vinegar

Resources: Get Started on Further Research   96

Dedication

This little book is dedicated to my Paternal Grandmother who we grandkids affectionately called 'Little Nana'. The 'little' came about due to her comparatively small size when compared to my Maternal Grandmother, who wasn't very tall, but was rather round.

Little Nana grew up surrounded by the common use of herbs in rural Scotland. I remember her telling me that as a child her mother would send her into the woods to collect various herbs and plants to be used for different purposes - both culinary and medicinally.

I also remember Little Nana showing me a small, tatty, leather bound copy of Culpeppers Herbal that she referenced fairly regularly. (I inherited that little book from her after she died). She told me how she would drink Sage tea to benefit her brain, and also how she took garlic in hot milk from time to time. She confessed that on more than one occasion she had used too much of the garlic, and when she did that the skin on the palms of her hands and the soles of her feet peeled!

Little Nana lived until she was 3 months away from her 100th birthday even though she smoked cigarettes until she was eighty, and I'm certain that she'd have lived well past 100 years if she'd stuck with the herbs, and stayed away from the doctors and their drugs. But sadly, as so many do, she succumbed to the mainstream allopathic medicine in her old age.

However even though she's gone, you'll read in this little book how my interest in herbs and then natural health originated from our conversations, and about some timely advice that my Little Nana gave me for which I am eternally grateful.

Chapter 1
How It All Started

BEFORE I GET STARTED, I'd like to explain who I am and how I came to be writing this book. I'm Mum to two (now adult) kids and Grandma to a couple of awesome grandchildren.

I've also been a Remedial Massage Therapist for close to 15 years at the time of writing this book and did some studying toward a degree in Naturopathy a few years ago, but never completed it. This was mainly because I realised it wasn't going to give me what I knew I wanted in life. However even though I quit the degree, I've continued to study, learn and experiment with all sorts of natural health topics over the years and I'm still a keen student today.

My interest in natural health eventuated from the simple fact that I became somewhat disenchanted with allopathic medicine, mainstream doctors, and their drugs, many, many years ago and the story of how this all came about goes something like this...

Once upon a time, I had a few health problems that had plagued me for *more* than a few years. When I look back in time, the problems that I had (predominantly digestive issues), were present most of my young life and became worse as a young adult. No matter how many doctors I went to, or how many of their pills I took, I really got no results. I was getting nowhere close to resolving my health problems.

During this time, my dear 'Little Nana' suggested to me that I should be taking Slippery Elm Bark to help with my ongoing digestive issues.

"What on earth is Slippery Elm Bark?" I asked her.

I'd never heard of the stuff and to be honest, I wasn't too keen to try it (I was somewhat less adventurous back then than I am today). But with the conviction of someone who knows what's good for them (and me), she quickly produced a packet from her pantry and proceeded to make me a drink from heated milk mixed with this 'slippery elm bark' powder.

Unconvinced, I tentatively took a sip once the mixture inside the cup was cool enough to drink and I remember instantly deciding that this stuff was 'yuck', quickly tipping the rest down the sink much to Little Nana's amusement. At the time (as young people are renowned for doing), I foolishly discarded her advice as some sort of old fashioned nonsense!

However a little over a year later after we had moved to Australia, and when the latest advice and the drug from the doctor had failed miserably, I remembered back to what my wise Little Nana had said, and in sheer desperation I decided to give the Slippery Elm Bark a go. I found a shop that sold it (which was not so easy back then as it is today), and I began to take it daily - initially in capsule form and eventually in the powdered version (which tends to be much more effective).

The good news is that slippery elm bark worked for me! I got relief from my symptoms with the slippery elm bark. Much more so than anything I'd had from the various doctors over the years, and as they say, the rest is history. I've never looked back.

My interest in herbs and how to use them grew from that initial success with slippery elm, and following that my interest in food and nutrition, my venture into bodywork and my passion for all things to do with natural health and healing.

And I love nothing more than to share what I've learned with anyone who will listen.

So I wanted to put this little book together for you to use at home with your family. This book is designed with beginners in mind that are looking for better ways to gain some control over their health and the health of their families.

I wanted to share some simple information, in an easy to understand way, that can help you begin that journey. Ideas that will allow you to take more control of your health and to stop relying so much on drugs that, let's face it, can not only be extremely damaging to your health with many side effects, but also, that more and more of us are realising simply don't work!

These essential home remedies are the beginning of a way that you can stop feeling so trapped and hopeless. So dependent on your doctor or pharmacist. They provide a way that will help rid you of the feeling that you've got no other choice but to have blind faith in your doctor. These simple remedies are a way to save you some of the money that you're probably spending on doctors visits, drugs and medicines that don't make you healthy, and that are in fact undermining your health and setting you up for more ill health in the future just by their very use.

The herbs, essential oils and other remedies contained herein are my favourites. They have been for many, many years. These are the simple remedies that I always keep on hand. These are the remedies that I rely on and use regularly (some more than others) to help keep me and mine well. These are my simple remedies that I have turned to again and again to over the past 20 years, and that I use either regularly to help prevent illness and maintain my health, or that I use to help recover my health when the need arises.

I sincerely hope that you take and use this information. Don't make the same mistake that I made when I discarded my Little Nana's advice! Don't just read this book and then not use the information that you've read. Put even a few of these ideas into practice and I'm sure you'll be happy that you did. These remedies are all simple. They're easy, some are free or (at least affordable) and when used correctly will move you closer to good health - not away from it as pharmaceutical medicines do!

I've done my best to make this book as short and sweet, and easy to read as possible. I've added basic information that I know from experience can make a difference every day.

There are many more ways that the herbs and remedies contained in this little book can be used, and my advice to you the reader is to get curious.

Once you've finished reading my ideas, don't leave it there. Do some more research on these remedies and others. The answers to your health challenges are all out there just waiting to be discovered!

My hope is that this book provides you with a *start*, and that it spurs you on to seek more information as my experience with Slippery Elm Bark did for me. The world needs more people with practical day to day knowledge of natural remedies.

Natural home remedies and their uses are truly a worthwhile topic in which to gain some knowledge. Home remedies can help to make you more able to take care of your own health and that's a wonderful thing. To be able to keep your family healthier is truly priceless. And to be able to share your knowledge to help others is a blessing.

Always remember that life without health is not life in its truest sense, but mere existence! Enjoy!

Chapter 2

The Digestive Healer: Slippery Elm

ULMUS RUBRA

Other names known by: Slippery Elm Bark; Red Elm; Indian Elm

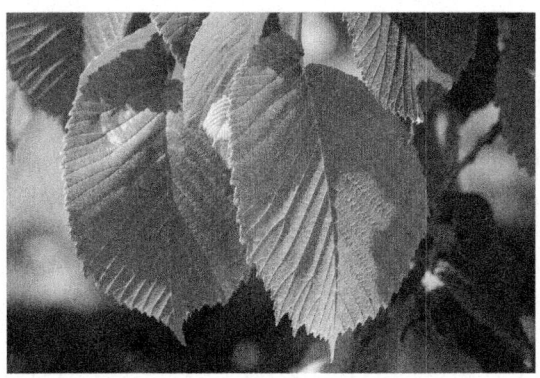

As you read in my introduction, Slippery Elm Bark was the beginning of my interest in herbs. This amazing remedy was introduced to me by my dear old Nana (who passed away in 2008, about 3 months before her 100 birthday). At the time (when she first recommended it) I was suffering with a lot of stomach and digestive problems. I was in and out of hospital, back and forth to doctors, with no real answers or solutions. Just different vague verdicts, and prescriptions that didn't work, from the many doctors and specialists I saw.

Even as a child my parents had me at the doctor on a regular basis with 'tummy problems' which were usually put down to constipation. I now realise that meant that the good old family Doctor really had no idea what was going on, and so the result of these consultations were that we usually left the doctors office with some prescription that didn't make any difference to my problems at all.

Once I got into my late teens and early 20's, the 'tummy troubles' got much worse, with frequent repeated visits to doctors and hospitals, tests and medications that still left me none the wiser and with no real changes.

I had ignored dear old Nana's advice until a few months after moving to Australia, when I discovered that once again the latest medication didn't work. I'd had enough of the doctors, their drugs, the poking and prodding and the tests, and so thinking about what Nana had told me, I went hunting for some slippery elm bark.

I had nothing to lose.

I figured I might as well try it as a last resort, and as I said already, the rest is history.

What Is Slippery Elm?

Slippery Elm is a powder made from the inner bark of the Red Elm tree. Slippery Elm was introduced to Western herbal medicine many years ago by the American Indians who used it throughout their history. It can now commonly be purchased in its powdered form, or in capsules or tablets.

I have found the powdered form to be the best option. It is the most effective way to take or use slippery elm as well as being the most cost effective, with the capsules being the next best option. The tablets often don't seem to be quite as effective probably due to the binders used to hold the tablets together making the slippery elm less available.

Slippery Elm has so many uses! The most common use being for problems in the digestive tract where it works brilliantly. Slippery Elm Bark is a very healing herb. It's mucilaginous quality soothes and assists with healing all tissues it comes into contact with, both internally and externally.

Taken internally, slippery elm can bring fast relief to indigestion. In my case, my eventual diagnosis all those years ago was dyspepsia (not that that really means anything) and a possible ulcer which was never confirmed. Slippery elm taken regularly, helped to heal and calm these problems, and then changes in my diet over the years eventually eliminated many of my digestive issues completely. However, I do still have a bit of a sensitive belly and so I still take slippery elm off and on. It always helps - every time.

Slippery elm is great for diarrhea as well as constipation. It will help with any issues, at any point along the digestive tract - from the mouth at the top, right down to the bottom! (Pardon the pun….).

Slippery Elm is not 'just a medicinal herb'. It is actually a food. It contains vitamins and minerals and has good nutritional value. I have read that Slippery Elm has been used by cancer patients on chemotherapy, and has been the only thing that they have been able to keep down, providing these patients with some good quality healing nutrition. It can be made into a gruel or porridge, and is great for invalids and those recovering from serious illness.

My Nana apparently used slippery elm in my Dad's bottle when he was a baby to settle his tummy. I wish I'd known about it when my kids were babies!

I have used it for our dog when she was a puppy. She had a very easily upset belly due to being taken from her mother at birth and bottle fed. We gave her slippery elm on her food every day for the first 12 months of her life, and now at 9 years old the overwhelming evidence seems to indicate that she has a cast iron gut!

Slippery Elm taken internally will help with coughs and other lung complaints, and it also supports the adrenal glands.

It can be used externally as a poultice for anything that is inflamed, or that needs drawing such as splinters or boils. I have used it just a week ago on a boil that my husband had had for about 3 weeks that wasn't clearing up. I made a poultice from approximately one teaspoon of slippery elm powder, a couple of drops of lavender oil and enough unpasteurised apple cider vinegar to form a paste. I put it on a gauze pad, wrapped a bandage around it, and left it on overnight. One application was all that was required. The boil cleared up over the next few days.

I also used the same mixture a few months ago on a spider bite. I didn't think to use it until about two days after the bite occurred behind my knee.

By this stage my leg from the knee down was very swollen, the area around the bite was hard and red, and very hot to touch, as well as being extremely uncomfortable. The first poultice made it feel a lot better within a few hours (although I felt quite sick and a little light headed for a while).

I left the poultice on over night, and by the morning the heat was gone along with a lot of the swelling. From memory I think I applied two fresh poultices over the next day and night, and it was good. The immediate area around the bite site was a little itchy for a while, and the skin peeled but I've never had any more problems with it.

The same can't be said for a previous bite from about a year ago that I had on my shoulder which was left untreated as I didn't realise it was a spider bite at the time it happened. This bite now still flares up and gets itchy and sore every couple of months. Maybe I should try the poultice next time it flares up and see if it helps to get rid of it!

How To Take Slippery Elm

To take slippery elm powder internally, mix about a teaspoon of the powder with a small amount of water and drink. If you leave it to sit for a while it will thicken and become mucilaginous (like wallpaper paste). It is great to take it like that, but if you can't handle it that thick, just mix and swallow before it thickens up. It'll still do a great job!

You can also use hot water to make a 'tea'. One teaspoon of slippery elm powder to a cup of hot water. This too will thicken up, but it usually provides quick results in cases of diarrhea or tummy upsets.

Adding a teaspoon of unpasteurised apple cider vinegar to your slippery elm mixture can also be beneficial for digestive issues.

So there we go. That's some basic info on my favorite herb Slippery Elm Bark. Buy some and keep it in the cupboard (it keeps forever), but don't forget it's there - use it!

How Do I Use Slippery Elm?

Use slippery elm for any, and all digestive issues such as irritable bowel, stomach pain, indigestion etc. Take it daily or multiple times a day if necessary.

Take slippery elm internally for coughs and lung complaints.

Make a poultice from slippery elm to draw and heal. Use for splinters, boils, or abscesses.

Use a slippery elm poultice for insect and spider bites.

Chapter 3
A Natural Antibiotic: Garlic

ALLIUM SATIVUM

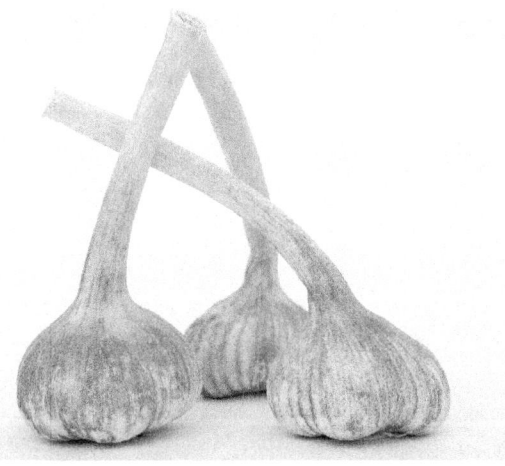

Garlic is probably best known to most of us as the pungent herb added to all sorts of dishes to impart its wonderful flavour, along with its pungent (but delicious) odour left on the breath.

Garlic will grow in good soil, and is easy to grow as its cultivation is pretty much 'plant and forget'. Plant garlic in the autumn, and harvest when the flowers die down. It can be grown in pots also. There are many varieties of Garlic available that include different flavours and sizes. Just make sure you choose a good tasting variety. Buy some different varieties from an organic shop, or your local farmers market, and try them out.

When buying garlic from the supermarket or grocery shop do be wary. The cheap, pure white Chinese garlic is best avoided. You can tell it by its colour and the fact that the roots are chopped off. The Chinese garlic that is commonly imported into our countries is apparently sprayed with chemicals that have been banned in other countries because they are harmful to humans. Plus there is a good chance that it's also irradiated. Unfortunately it is also the cheapest and most common garlic available here in Australia. Some supermarket chains sell *only*

Chinese garlic, so be warned - hunting for a better option might necessary!

The best way to use garlic is in your food - every day if possible! I use it in most dishes that I cook, and I try to use it raw as often as possible. Use it raw in things such as garlic butter, dressings, aioli, guacamole, hummus and fresh vegetable juices.

I use it sometimes by scraping a raw clove over hot toasted sourdough bread, and then spread the bread with avocado, and add salt and pepper. It's delicious!

If you worry about the smell of garlic on your breath just chew on some parsley afterwards as it gets rid of the smell apparently. I personally don't tend to worry too much. I've smelt much worse smells on peoples breath than garlic, and for a garlic lover, the smell is not offensive at all, but rather delicious instead!

I also make guacamole, or my version of it. My version of guacamole is truly simple and requires only crushed garlic, avocado, salt and pepper. Just mash it up and voila! It's done.

Note: when I say <u>salt</u> I'm of course talking about <u>pink Himalayan salt</u> or unprocessed <u>Celtic salt</u> - not the pure white, mineral deficient, processed sodium chloride found in the supermarkets!

Garlic has incredible properties. It is a natural broad spectrum antibiotic that your body does not appear to build up a resistance to, which means its antibiotic effect continues over time to help keep you healthy. Garlic kills bacteria, viruses and fungus, as well as intestinal worms. It has been shown to lower LDL cholesterol and triglycerides, while increasing the *good* HDL cholesterol levels. It also removes heavy metals such as lead from the blood as well as preventing accumulation in the first place. It helps to lower blood pressure, and is used by some cultures to help control diabetes.

Garlic boosts the immune system which in turn helps to prevent many illnesses from the common cold to cancer. Many studies point to garlic's anti-tumour effects, with one study showing residents in an area of China who don't eat garlic having a whopping <u>1000 times</u> the rate of stomach cancer, than those in a neighboring area where garlic was consumed regularly. (Stomach cancer is one of the most common cancers found in China).

Garlic was used in both the first and second world wars to prevent gangrene in wounds. It is also used to treat conditions of the retina, hepatitis, and almost all lung conditions.

Garlic is a truly amazing herb and a must have in the kitchen! If you don't like it then do your best to learn to like it! Add a little to your food and build it up. That's what I've always done with things that I know are going to be good for me, but that I didn't initially like. Just keep at it and you'll learn to love it.

I've known people who take garlic every day by cutting it into smaller pieces and swallowing it whole like a pill. That can work. But it pays to remember that the cutting or crushing of the garlic is necessary as it changes the alliin to allicin, which is the active constituent.

Garlic also contains a good number of vitamins and minerals, as well as organic sulphur, which are all essential to our health.

A slice of garlic placed over a wart and covered with a band aid, and then replaced regularly will help to get rid of the wart.

Garlic (along with some other natural products) can cause 'problems' with some medications. An example of this that is specific to garlic, is blood thinning medications. However to me, it seems that the problem is not with the garlic, but the medication. Doesn't it make sense to use something natural, and health promoting (like garlic) to thin your blood if necessary, rather than expensive, toxic medication with its side effects? Speak to your doctor, and if necessary get him or her to monitor what's happening and do what makes sense to you - with regard for your doctors advice of course!

The occasional person may be allergic, or sensitive to garlic. Too much garlic can cause indigestion in some people, and can irritate the skin in a few sensitive individuals. But don't let that keep you from using this wonderful herb if possible. Your body will thank you for it.

How Do I Use Garlic?

Take garlic for colds and flu, or any time you need to boost your immune system.

Want to avoid antibiotics? Garlic can help.

Use a slice of garlic to get rid of warts and plantar warts by putting a slice over the wart and keeping it there with a plaster or bandage.

Use garlic in cooking for general health.

Cut garlic into pieces, crush slightly and swallow whole as you would a pill or capsule.

Chapter 4
Lose Weight & Lower Blood Pressure With Chili

CAPSICUM SPECIES

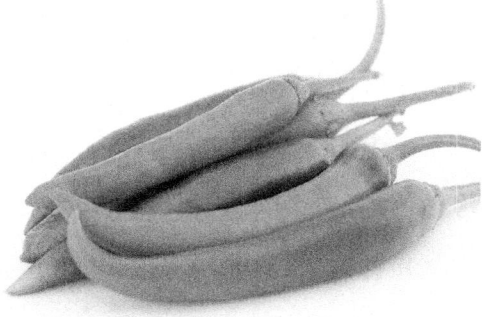

Chilies (sometimes spelled Chilli with two l's) are hot stuff and they're amazing!

Don't these herbs just keep get better and better?

Chilies originated in Mexico and central North America, and evidence indicates that they have been used since 7000BC. That's a long time! They were introduced into Asia in the 16th century and became part of the staple diet in Asian countries.

Chilies are easily grown from seed, or alternatively you can buy plants or seedlings at a local market or a nursery if they're available in your area. Chili plants can either be grown in the ground, or they also grow easily in pots. They aren't too keen on frost, so if you live in a frosty area, move them to a sheltered spot when the frosts are around.

And if you have a dog that eats literally anything like our old Bull Mastiff Nala, you might have to hide them from the dog. We were blaming the birds for stealing our very hot chilies from our chili bush, only to discover that it was actually the dog stealing them as they were ripening up!

Bizarre but true….

Chilies are a bit like garlic in that they've been used for almost as long as humans have been eating.

These spicy fruits share with Garlic the ability to have huge health benefits on all parts of the body. Chilies help to keep us strong and healthy, boosting the immune system and making us feel great.

Chili works as a pain killer in the body and has been shown to help with headache and migraine. It is used in salves and ointments which are used externally to treat the pain of arthritis and other pain.

Chili is a well-known and well researched anti-cancer herb, and it, like garlic, helps to lower blood pressure, keep your heart healthy and is even thought to boost metabolism helping those consuming chili to lose or control their weight!

Chili has been shown to reduce inflammation in the body and in the digestive tract, and it can help to kill the bacteria that causes stomach ulcers.

Again, like garlic, use it in your cooking whenever possible. Fresh is best or use dried chili if the fresh fruits are not available. There are many different varieties of chili with differing flavours and some are *definitely* hotter than others.

Experiment and find a variety you like. A word of warning though, they *are* addictive, and over time the taste buds tend to grow to like it hotter and hotter if you consume chili regularly. That's not a bad thing however, as chilies truly are an awesome food and full of vitamins A and C.

How Do I Use Chili?

My husband has recently become a chili fan after quitting smoking. It's interesting what happens with the taste buds once you quit the cigarettes. Prior to quitting he couldn't handle any chili at all and complained bitterly if I even put a sniff of it in his meal!

Now he can't get enough of the stuff. He has even been known of late to add fresh chili to his coffee (in the plunger) from time to time. I must admit, it adds a nice kick so long as it's not too much.

I use chilies mostly in cooking - sauces, soups, stews, stir fries - pretty much anything really.

I add chili or cayenne to herbal teas sometimes also. Once again it gives a healthy kick!

Use chili raw in salads without the seeds (the seeds are the hottest part of the chili) or scorch the skins over a flame or in the grill and then remove the skins and seeds to create a sweet, hot treat to add to a salad, or over a nice piece of steak.

I have also read of people using Habenero Chilies (one of the hottest chilies you can get) on toast, along with grated raw ginger, to combat cancer. If you do a Google search, you'll find information on people using this treatment (I personally have never needed to try this and I'm hoping that with my regular consumption of these herbs along with a healthy lifestyle I won't ever have to).

Some people find that chili soaked in olive oil or coconut oil for a week or more and used on arthritis or painful joints is beneficial.

Chapter 5
The Healer: Aloe Vera

ALOE BARBADENSIS

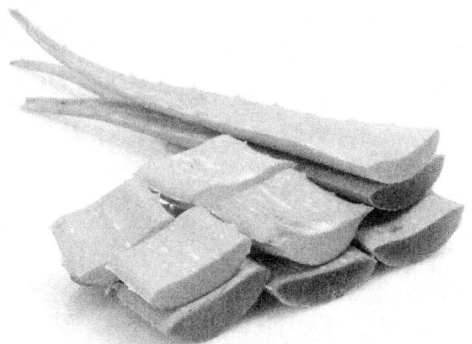

Aloe Vera originates from East Africa and is a very easy plant to grow. In fact, Aloe Vera pretty much thrives on neglect. I find it best to grow it in a pot, or somewhere where it is easy to contain, because if it likes the growing conditions, it will multiply and spread readily!

Aloe Vera is sometimes confused with Agave, or other succulents that don't have the same properties as the true Aloe Vera because they look similar. However, once you're familiar with what Aloe Vera looks like, you'll find that you don't confuse it with anything else.

Aloe has a long history of use, and research has shown it to have incredible healing powers when used both internally and externally.

Aloe can be used for many skin problems. It will assist the healing of wounds and will relieve itching. It is incredibly soothing, and when used topically it helps with burns, including sunburn, where its application is cooling, soothing, and refreshing. It can be said that if it hurts, stings, itches or burns put aloe vera on it.

I even discovered that fresh aloe vera gel relieves the burning pain that is caused by rubbing the eyes or face after cutting up chilies... This is something that I seem to do regularly, and it doesn't matter how often I do it I just don't learn so this discovery was very welcome!

To use aloe vera externally, just break a leaf off and cut it open. Apply the fresh gel found inside the leaf by wiping it over the skin.

Used internally, both research and practical application has proved aloe to be most useful in digestive issues, where again it is extremely healing, calms inflammation and gives relief to many complaints.

Make Your Own Aloe Vera Juice

Aloe vera juice can be easily prepared at home for internal use. Simply remove the clear gel from the outside leaf. Rinse the gel under running water or place in fresh water to remove as much of the yellow latex as possible. It is advisable to remove the yellow sap (latex) found close to the outer part of the leaf as it can cause cramping and diarrhea. Place the clear gel in a blender with filtered water and a little lemon juice (optional) and blend well. Refrigerate and drink regularly. Aloe Vera juice is refreshing and soothing to the digestive system.

Used internally, Aloe has anti-cancer properties (isn't it exciting that these herbs are all known to help prevent cancer?). Studies have also shown aloe to be of great benefit in cases of AIDs where it has been used regularly.

Aloe Vera has shown to be of benefit for indigestion, asthma, arthritis, diabetes, liver problems, hemorrhoids, urinary tract infections, prostate problems and much, much more.

Note: Too much aloe vera can cause digestive disturbance and also avoid taking this herb internally during menstruation if you have trouble with heavy bleeding as it may make your bleeding heavier.

How Do I Use Aloe Vera?

I use Aloe externally by applying the fresh gel found inside the leaf to sunspots, sunburn, skin problems, itches, bites etc.

Been cutting up chili? Use fresh aloe vera gel on your eyes if you get chili in them from your hands. It really helps fast!

I have used aloe inside my ears to give relief from itchy ears by applying the aloe gel with a cotton bud.

I've also used it also to get rid of warts. Aloe vera applied to warts and verrucas daily will eventually get rid of them (it can take a while but stick at it. If you forget a day or two, it doesn't matter, just keep at it).

Make your own Aloe Vera juice and drink it regularly.

Aloe vera is an herb that once in your garden, can be there for life, waiting to be needed which I find is often once you're in the habit of using it.

CHAPTER 6

From Cancer to Morning Sickness: Ginger

ZINGIBER OFFICINALE

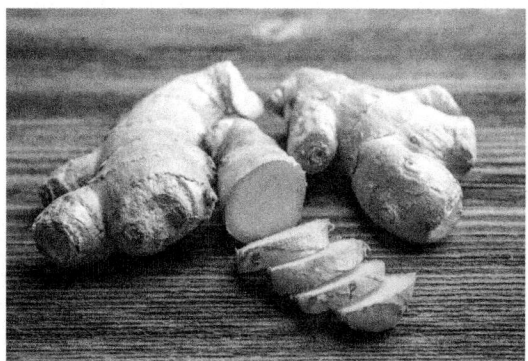

Ginger originates from South-East Asia and has been cultivated for so long, that it is apparently no longer found growing wild. The part used is the root of the plant, and it gives the zing to Asian dishes and Indian chutneys.

The Chinese consider ginger an important herb to treat colds, and to encourage sweating. Ginger is also very effective for treating digestive disorders such as gas and nausea. Due to its effect on reducing nausea, it is widely used to prevent motion sickness as well as the common morning sickness experienced by so many women during pregnancy.

Ginger is warming, which makes it useful to get rid of a fever, as well as stimulating the circulation. The essential oil is wonderful when used in massage oil, as it is great for producing heat, and increasing circulation in sore muscles.

If you'd like to buy essential oils, see the resources at the end of this book.

Ginger also has anti-cancer properties (yet another one) and has been used in alternative cancer treatments. It has, of course, been used as previously mentioned, with habanero chilies to treat cancer. It also helps to reduce inflammation in the body.

How Do I Use Ginger?

I use ginger a lot in my cooking, chopped finely or grated, in any Asian style dish or stir fry.

I also use ginger in a tea regularly. It's so easy to make. Simply slice some ginger, put it in a cup and fill with boiling water.

A tea made with fresh ginger and licorice root is a delicious combination. It combines the heat and pungency of the ginger with the sweetness of the licorice root to make a delicious, relaxing, and healthy drink that can be enjoyed hot or cold. (Note: Those with high blood pressure should avoid licorice root as it can exacerbate the condition).

I sometimes also combine licorice root with Fennel Seed which makes another great tasting tea that calms the belly and gets rid of flatulence (always handy...). This combination is a great alternative to the licorice root for those with blood pressure issues. Fennel seed is also reputed to help with weight loss.

Ginger tea is great for morning sickness and motion sickness.

If I ever feel like I may be getting a cold, I make a tea with fresh ginger, thyme, lemon juice and rind, honey and sometimes some garlic or cayenne. Mmmmmmm! Those cold bugs don't stand a chance!

Tip: When you make these teas, either make them in a teapot with a lid or if making in a cup, place a dish or plate on the top of the cup for a few minutes while the tea infuses. This helps to keep the oils from the herbs in the tea and to stops them from evaporating out with the steam. This will help to make your teas more beneficial.

Chapter 7
Thyme For Coughs and Colds

THYMUS VULGARIS

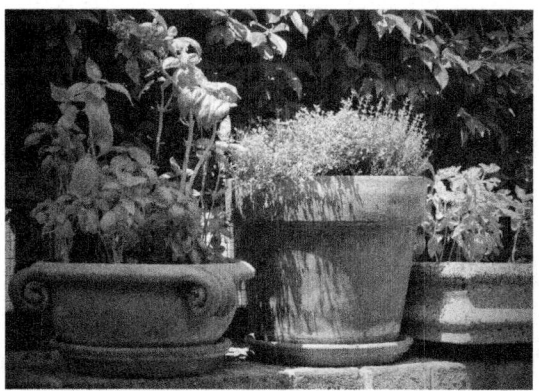

Thyme is a creeping ground cover with small white to lilac flowers. It has small oval leaves that come to a point, is very fragrant and grows to 30cm high and 30cm wide.

This tough little ground cover will grow almost anywhere. It grows naturally from the West Mediterranean to Southwest Italy where it grows on dry rocky soil. Give Thyme a sunny spot and it will generally flourish. Thyme can be propagated from seed, but I have always found the easiest way is to dig up a piece with some roots and transplant it. Do it away from frosts, but still when the weather is cool and the soil damp to give it time to establish before the heat of summer.

There are apparently over 200 different species of thyme, and there is often confusion when it comes to identifying them even in nurseries. All varieties are all suitable for use in cooking, with some having quite different flavors such as Lemon Thyme and Caraway Thyme.

I use thyme often in cooking. I use it in soups, stews, and pasta sauces. Thyme has a great flavor and when used regularly, will help to keep you, and those you cook for, stay healthy.

As a rough guide, if I were cooking a sauce for four people, I'd pick and use a couple of tablespoons (once chopped) depending on how many other herbs I'm using with it. I often use Rosemary and Sage, along with Garlic and a bit of Chili. Chop the thyme up finely, removing any woody stalks. The thin, soft branches that chop up easily are usually okay to leave in.

Use Thyme For Coughs

Thyme is amazing for coughs! This is where it stands out above anything else I've ever come across. It has been used to treat coughs throughout history, including whooping cough and bronchitis. Thyme is great for clearing congestion.

Thymol (considered to be the effective constituent in thyme) is used in many pharmaceutical cough syrups. However as is always the case, 'the whole is greater than the sum of its parts'. This means that by extracting the Thymol, removing it from the rest of the constituents contained in the herb, and then adding other not so healthy ingredients such as sugar, colours and who knows what else to create the end product, the commercial cough syrups generally remain only marginally effective if at all.

Nature really is <u>much smarter</u> and provides us with these little bundles of parts, wrapped up as a whole, in the perfect combinations to be used by us, and to be effective at increasing health.

I first got an inkling into Thyme and its use for coughs many years ago when my daughter, as a young child, used to suffer terribly with a persistent cough that appeared each time she had a bit of a cold. This cough would often continue for months after the cold was gone.

Her cough would keep her awake at night and would also concern the schoolteachers so much that they would phone us to come and get her even though she was not 'sick' as such, but because she would cough until she gagged.

The doctor, convinced that it was asthma, prescribed every manner of asthma preventative, puffer, and inhaler that he could but none made the slightest difference.

We had tried all the cough syrups, mixtures, and anything else we came across. This continued for a few years until we tried Thyme tea. The Thyme didn't stop her getting the cough, but it did stop her from coughing, allowed her to sleep, and generally cleared up her cough in a few days rather than months! She hated drinking the stuff, but eventually she realized that it did work and so she took it happily. I used to send her to school with a drink bottle full of Thyme tea so she could have some during the day, which she happily did.

Thyme is also great as a gargle for gum disease and throat infections. It has shown to be effective against the shingles virus (herpes zoster), it helps digestion, may help with menstrual cramps, and can help destroy parasites.

How Do I Use Thyme?

To make the Thyme tea, simply pick about a tablespoon of leaves and stalks, put in a small teapot, or cup and fill with boiling water. Cover the cup to keep the steam in for about 5 minutes and it's ready to go. Easy as that!

If you don't like the taste as it is, add some fresh lemon juice and a teaspoon of raw honey. It's delicious! This tea can be used also at the onset of a cold. I find that it'll usually stop it in its tracks. For this purpose, I usually add some fresh ginger as well as the lemon and honey - even some Cayenne Pepper! If I feel like I'm coming down with something, I'll have one before bed then see how I feel in the morning. If I still feel a little like it might be there (or often even if it doesn't) I'll have another in the morning. No virus or bug is going to beat that combination!

The great thing is that you can have Thyme tea as much as you like because it's only going to do your body good.

An alternative to fresh thyme is to use Thyme essential oil. This oil can be rubbed on the chest and/or the soles of the feet, but always make sure you dilute Thyme oil with a carrier oil (eg coconut oil). Thyme essential oil is a *hot* oil and will irritate the skin if used neat!

To buy Thyme essential oil see the resources at the end of this book.

CHAPTER 8

The Master Alkaliser: Lemon

CITRUS LIMON

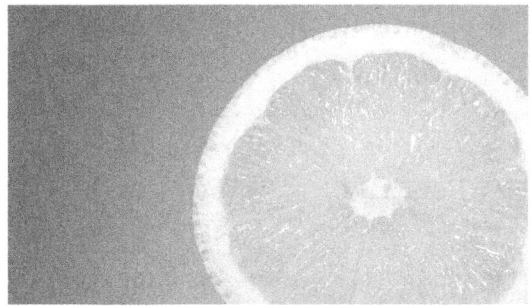

We all know lemons. They're the sour, yellow fruit that we squeeze over our fish, right?

As common as this fruit is, the truth is that it's underutilized, undervalued and very useful for keeping us healthy!

Lemons are easily grown. Once you get a lemon tree established, either in the garden or in a large tub, it will probably keep you in lemons all year round. They are a beautiful tree with glossy leaves that for part of the year, get covered in white citrus blossoms with a gorgeous citrus smell!

Lemon juice taken in water each day is probably one of the simplest things you can do for your health. I do it off and on, but really should keep it up.

Although lemons are acidic, once in your body they become alkaline. Lemon water is useful for bloating, indigestion and heartburn, arthritis, gout, and it will assist the bowels to eliminate waste efficiently helping with both constipation *and* diarrhea.

The lemon is a wonderful herb for the liver and is thought to help dissolve gallstones. It helps those who have problems with bleeding disorders and excessive menstruation.

Lemon is great in cases of colds, flu, for coughs, asthma, and sore throats.

Lemons are a real health tonic. There are apparently scientific reasons as to why the humble lemon is so effective, and it is apparently to do with cations and anions, but I won't attempt to go into that. Suffice it to say that everyone could do with a little lemon each day.

Remember always use <u>fresh</u> lemon juice - not the bottled stuff!

How Do I Use Lemon?

I use Lemon in herbal teas sometimes. For example I might combine it with thyme, ginger, and some honey.

I often have a little lemon squeezed into hot water first thing in the morning. That's a great habit to get into!

I often use lemon and its peel when I make fresh juices.

During our hot summers we drink a lot of sparkling mineral water. Each afternoon we sit in the sun with a glass of icy cold mineral water with lemon squeezed into it - just lovely!

Note that Limes have the same properties and can be used instead of lemons.

CHAPTER 9
From Breast Milk to Farts: Fennel Seed

FOENICULUM VULGARE

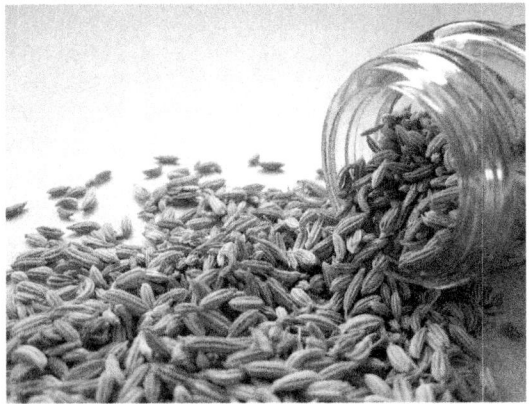

Fennel is the tall feathery looking plant that is commonly seen growing as a weed on the side of the road, and on wasteland type areas in temperate climates. It looks similar to, and can be mistaken for Dill.

Fennel bulbs are commonly seen in the vegetable section of the supermarket these days, and gradually this herb is becoming a little more known as a vegetable. It has a strong licorice flavour and can be used raw in salads or cooked as a hot vegetable.

It has long been suggested that consuming fennel helps with weight loss, and it is an effective diuretic. Fennel seed is very effective at calming the digestive system, relieving flatulence, and other digestive issues such as indigestion, constipation, and diarrhea. It was one of the ingredients in the 'Gripe Water' that we used to give to our babies to relieve colic.

Fennel seed promotes the production and flow of milk in breast feeding Mums with the properties of the fennel passing through to the milk, helping to prevent colicky babies.

It also works for animals such as goats, and fennel is often used to boost milk production by canny goat farmers!

Other uses for fennel include menstruation problems, anemia, respiratory problems, and eye problems.

How Do I Use Fennel?

Occasionally I buy fennel bulb and use it in cooking or salads, but after doing some research for this book, I think I'll start buying it more often and juice it!

I mostly use the seeds. I use them in soups and stews for flavouring, and to impart their wonderful assistance with digestion. I use the seeds to make tea quite often. Of late I combine them with fresh ginger. It makes a wonderful relaxing and refreshing tea. Simply slice some fresh ginger. Put in a cup along with about half a teaspoon of fennel seed. Fill with boiling water. Cover for a few minutes to keep in the steam and the volatile oils, then drink.

The seeds can also be chewed after meals to aid digestion and settle the belly.

Fennel essential oil can be beneficial for the same reasons as the whole seed. It can be used internally for digestion and to assist with weightloss.

If you wish to use essential oils internally, ensure that you buy a brand that is safe to consume. To buy pure, safe essential oils, see the link in the resources at the end of this book.

Chapter 10
Breath Deep and Be Calm with Lemon Balm

MELISSA OFFICINALIS

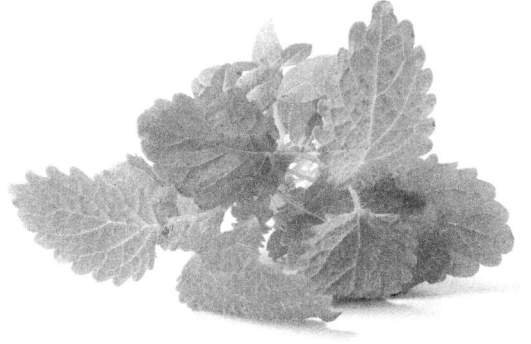

Lemon Balm (also known as Melissa) gets its common name due to its lemon fragrance. Lemon Balm is an attractive plant that grows well in pots as it prefers good drainage (wet ground can kill it). It's not keen on frost so keep it under cover during frosty weather. Lemon Balm self-seeds readily.

Lemon balm originates in the Mediterranean and has been cultivated for at least 2000 years.

The Muslim herbalist Avicenna recommended the herb 'to make the heart merry'.

It has been claimed that Lemon Balm can revitalize the whole body. John Hussey of Sydenham, who lived to the age of 116, breakfasted for fifty years on Lemon Balm tea sweetened with honey and this breakfast habit was shared by Llewelyn Prince of Glamorgan, who died in his 108th year!

When in flower it will attract bees in great numbers for, they obviously realise its value!

Lemon balm is a great herb for the nervous system. It is a tranquiliser. It calms a nervous stomach, colic, and heart spasms. The leaves are also reputed to lower blood pressure.

The actions of Lemon Balm are very gentle, as well as effective, and so it is often suggested for children and babies. Lemon balm lifts the spirits and is helpful in cases of depression, nervousness, and insomnia.

The tea quickly brings on a sweat that will help to combat fevers, colds and flu, and it has antiviral properties that have been shown to be effective against mumps, herpes (cold sores) and other viruses.

Because Melissa is used in Europe to treat Graves' disease (hyperthyroid) there is confusion about its effects on the thyroid, the assumption being that it only lowers production of thyroid hormones. However, it has also shown to raise thyroid hormone in cases of under active thyroid (hypothyroid) and so possibly works more as a 'balancer or regulator' of these hormones. Herbs generally do not work the way that drugs do by causing one specific reaction, they often work instead with our bodies to correct, balance, and heal.

Lemon balm boosts the immune system, stimulates the liver and gallbladder promoting detoxification, and has an energising effect on people with fatigue.

How Do I Use Lemon Balm?

I make tea with Lemon Balm. I simply pick a couple of sprigs, put it in a cup or teapot, and cover with boiling water. Sweeten with honey if desired (always raw honey - not pasteurised) and enjoy!

I also make lemon balm tincture using alcohol to extract the lemon balm. That way I always have some on hand and it can be used when needed. I made a video about how to do this.

You can see that video here: https://youtu.be/kzeFgUBe2dA

CHAPTER 11

The Swiss Army Knife: Lavender Essential Oil

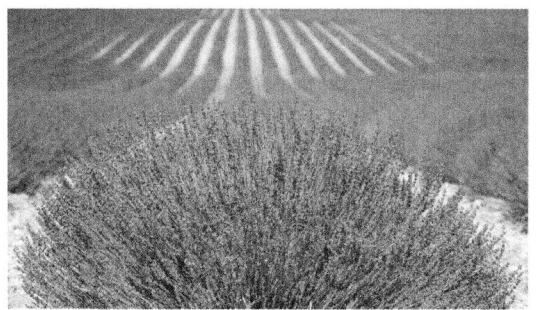

LAVENDER OIL IS A must have for the medicine cupboard. It is known as the 'Swiss army knife' of essential oils because it can be used for so many things! It's probably the safest and most well-known of all the essential oils and can be used undiluted on the skin.

Note: Always make sure you buy a good quality, pure 100% essential oil! Not a cheap fragrant oil or mixed oil. Lavender oil is commonly tainted, if it's really cheap, it's probably not pure and therefore unsuitable for use on your body! See the resources page at the end of this book.

Lavender oil is anti-fungal, anti-bacterial, anti-viral, soothing, restorative, healing, and just amazing stuff!

Emotional properties: Lavender oil is the oil of calm communication.

How Do I Use Lavender Essential Oil?

For Lavender oil I'm going to list just some of its uses. It has so many! I either have used it or still use it for the following:

- Massage - mix a few drops with a good quality cold pressed vegetable oil (Coconut, Olive, Sweet Almond, or Grapeseed) - make sure it's cold pressed though!

- Rub a little on the temples for headache

- Use straight on bites and stings - especially ant bites!

- As described earlier, mixed with slippery elm, and use as poultice for splinters, spider bites, boils - anything that requires drawing

- Applied straight for thrush - it burns a bit, but calms itching quickly, and I always found it got rid of that insane itching faster than pharmaceutical creams/treatments.

- Use Lavender undiluted on pimples

- Use it straight on cuts, wounds etc

- Put a drop on babies bedding and they will sleep soundly

- Use a few drops in the bath for relaxation, or in the kids' bath to get them to sleep faster

- Use on sunburn, burns and scalds. It is one of the absolute best treatments for burns (always seek medical advice for serious burns)

- Burn it in an oil burner or diffuse it in an electric diffuser. Lavender is relaxing and helps stop the spread of colds, flu etc.

- Use Lavender in ointments or in skin care

- Add it to natural hair treatments and products

There are so many uses for Lavender oil! I always pack it whenever we go away anywhere. It's definitely a must have.

Chapter 12
Breathe Easy with Peppermint Essential Oil

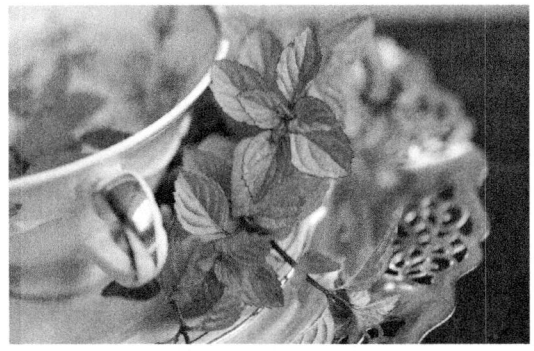

PEPPERMINT OIL IS USED a lot in commercial products such as dental products, sweets and more, both for its flavour and for its scent. It's a flavour that most people are familiar with and that many of us are partial to.

How Do I Use Peppermint Oil?

Peppermint oil can be taken internally by putting a few drops in a glass of water. Drink it for indigestion, upset stomach, flatulence, or low appetite.

It can also be diluted and applied to the forehead to relieve headache.

From my own experience, Peppermint essential oil surpasses all others for clearing the nose and congestion when suffering colds, sinus, or any time that the nose is congested for any reason. It can be easily used by putting a couple of drops on a tissue and inhaled, or it can be inhaled in steam by adding the oil to hot water and then covering the head and the bowl with a towel and inhaling in the vapours.

Used externally, peppermint oil helps to relieve pain and aids circulation.

Inhaling peppermint oil clears the head and makes you more alert. Burn it in the oil burner or diffuse it for its lovely minty fragrance and its head clearing effect.

Emotional properties: Peppermint oil is the oil of a buoyant heart.

Again, always ensure that you buy 100% essential oil and if you choose to use peppermint oil internally, only use a brand that is suited for internal use.

See resources at the end of this book.

Chapter 13

Used For Almost Everything: Apple Cider Vinegar

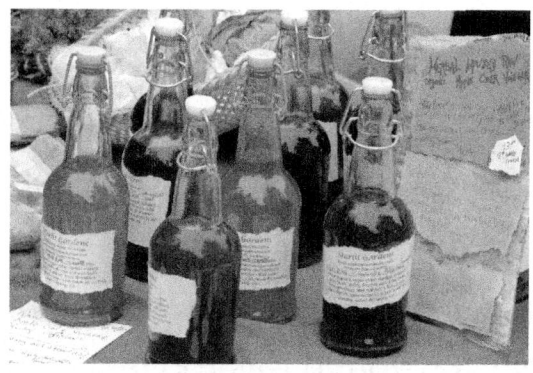

APPLE CIDER VINEGAR (OTHERWISE known as ACV) is another remedy that has more uses than I can list here. Do some research! It's amazing stuff.

Always buy raw, unpasteurised ACV (Apple Cider Vinegar) that contains the 'mother'.

You can tell it's the good stuff by looking through the bottle. It will have a cloudy sediment which is the 'mother' floating around the bottom of the bottle. If the ACV you're looking at is all clear and clean looking (as many of those that you find in the supermarket are), it's pasteurized and won't have the same health-giving effects.

Uses for ACV are many and varied. Of course, you can use ACV on salads and in dressings, but it can also be used in other ways.

How Do I Use Apple Cider Vinegar?

You can take ACV in water on a daily basis. The recommendation is 2 tablespoons daily added to water and sipped throughout the day (although some people take more). When I first started taking ACV, I personally found this too much for me every day as it seemed to upset my belly, so I started with only half a teaspoon to a teaspoon a day, and then gradually increased it. I now take two tablespoons in water every morning with no problems.

Taken in water it can help with weight loss. It also helps with tummy upsets, and it can be useful to take if you think you might have eaten something that's going to give you a dose of food poisoning! It can help to stop diarrhea also.

Add it to your pet's water to keep them healthy - they'll love you for it.

ACV can be used externally on skin complaints, and as I described earlier, I used it in my poultice with slippery elm and lavender oil with amazing success for my spider bite!

As I already said, do some more learning on this one - it's amazing the results some people get with ACV. Experiment for yourself and see how you go with it.

If you don't like the taste of ACV, a great tip is to mix it not only with water but add some liquid stevia and natural vanilla essence to sweeten.

ACV can be diluted and used to pour through the hair after washing to help with dandruff and scalp complaints. Use a couple of tablespoons diluted in a cup of water.

Add 1 teaspoon of ACV to slippery elm and water for digestive issues.

Chapter 14

From Gout To Cleaning: Baking Soda

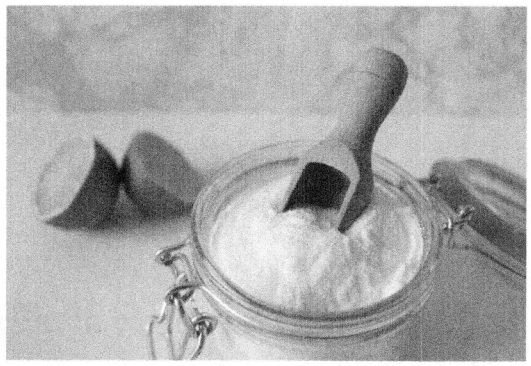

BICARBONATE OF SODA IS one of those simple remedies that was used commonly for all sorts of ailments in the past but has been almost forgotten by most people in this age of pharmaceutical drugs and scientific medicine.

Bicarbonate of Soda (otherwise known as bicarb or baking soda) is one of the remedies that my little Nana used to both recommend and use herself for an upset tummy or indigestion, and it works well.

First and foremost, make sure that when you buy baking soda to take internally you buy an aluminium free variety such as Bob's Red Mill. This comes as a bit of a shock to many people who don't realise that many brands carried in the supermarket chains may contain aluminium which means that while they're suitable for cleaning you really don't want to take them internally.

If you visit your local health food store, they're likely to carry a brand without aluminium, or at least be able to order one in for you if you ask.

Baking soda helps keep your body alkaline.

Keeping your body PH slightly on the alkaline side is known to be one of the factors that will help to keep you healthy. When the PH of your body is too acid, it can cause ill health and be a contributing factor to all sorts of diseases from cancer to arthritis.

Baking soda has been used for many years as a home remedy, as well as being used both historically and currently in the emergency rooms of hospitals around the world to save lives.

Baking soda can be used to help to keep your body more alkaline, and in fact its ability to alkalise is the reason it works so well for many of the ailments that it assists with. For example, when you take it for an upset tummy, that's why it works - it's combating the acidity in the digestive system that's causing the tummy upset or the heartburn.

Note: *Do not take baking soda after a very large meal when extremely full.*

Baking soda is often very helpful in cases of gout. It can apparently work quickly to relieve the terrible pain that gout causes. I have read testimonials from people who having been long time gout sufferers, and who have found that they can use baking soda to both prevent and relieve gout attacks successfully from the time that they come across this valuable information.

Baking Soda as A Cancer Treatment

There are a number of doctors around the world who are currently treating cancer patients with baking soda. Baking soda is apparently often used in oncology as an adjunct to chemotherapy treatment, and it is being used by an oncologist named Dr Simoncini in Italy to treat cancer patients with amazing success instead of chemotherapy. You can read more about Dr Simoncini's theories and his work with cancer in his book titled 'Cancer Is a Fungus: A Revolution in Tumor Therapy'. .

Another well-known doctor using baking soda to treat cancer and other diseases is Dr Mark Sircus. He has written an excellent and in-depth book on using baking soda for many health issues including cancer. You can find more about his book here: https://suewoledge.co.nz/favourite-books

Please note: It is highly recommended to test the PH level of your urine and saliva if using baking soda daily as being too alkaline can be life threatening. PH testing can be done using PH testing strips. For information on taking baking soda safely and contraindications visit Dr Sircus's website here: http://drsircus.com/medicine/sodium-bicarbonate-baking-soda/warnings-and-contraindications

Baking Soda for Odors Including Bad Breath

One of the best applications for baking soda is to get rid of odors - all sorts of odors - both in the house and from your body! A dish of baking soda in the fridge will help to stop smells lingering and used in drains it can help to remove bad smells.

Baking soda can also be used to clean teeth. That's right - just wet your toothbrush, dip the bristles in the baking soda and brush your teeth with it. Baking soda will neutralise odors and help to stop bad breath, as well as leaving your teeth feeling great. If you don't like the taste, do what I do and make your own natural toothpaste (or toothpowder) using baking soda and bentonite clay, but that is flavoured with essential oils and stevia to make it taste good!

Click to check out my Toothpowder Recipe here.

How To Take Baking Soda

Dissolve baking soda in a glass of water and drink it. (Warning! It's an acquired taste so be prepared.) Some people take baking soda daily but be aware that there are reports that the salt it contains may contribute to high blood pressure, and as already stated, you need to monitor your PH to ensure that you're not taking too much.

Chapter 15
More Handy Remedies

I'VE ADDED SOME ADDITIONAL remedies here that I use off and on, that I've found to be valuable additions to the medicine cabinet. I'm certain you will too.

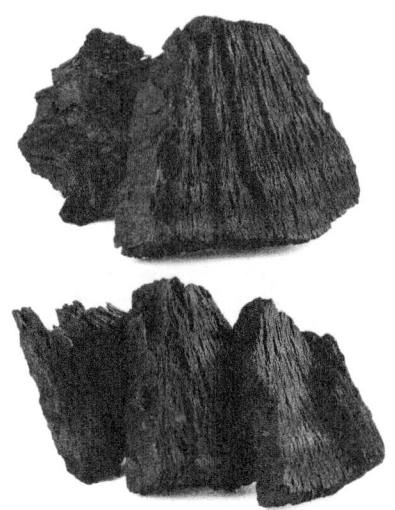

Activated Charcoal

Activated Charcoal is black, powdered charcoal that is usually made from coconut shell, and comes in powder, tablets, or capsules. Charcoal useful for belly problems, gas, diarrhea, constipation, indigestion etc.

Charcoal is also good for hangovers! This is a useful piece of information we discovered many years ago...

It is commonly used in emergency medicine as it is effective in absorbing some poisons. Charcoal can save lives when used correctly and taken in a sufficient amount. It is commonly used in A&E departments of hospitals and by veterinarians for patients that have been poisoned.

Charcoal is also useful for bad breath and body odour and can be purchased from health shops or online.

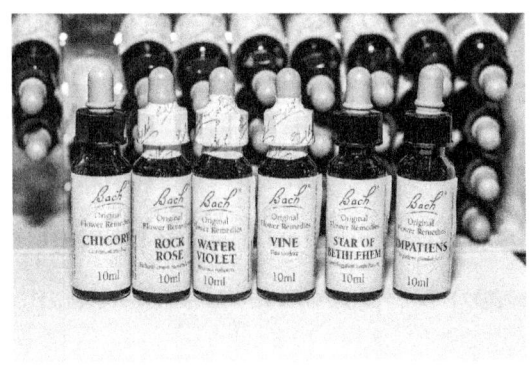

Bach Rescue Remedy

Bach Rescue Remedy is a flower remedy. Flower remedies are homeopathic type remedies created from specific flowers.

Rescue Remedy is useful for both humans and animals, during times of nervousness, stress, fear or anxiety. It can also be used in times of bereavement, relationship breakdowns, shock, accident/emergency etc.

Rescue Remedy is completely safe for all ages and is a very handy remedy to always have on hand. I carry a bottle in my handbag and have done for many years.

This too can be purchased from health shops, online and from some Naturopathic physicians.

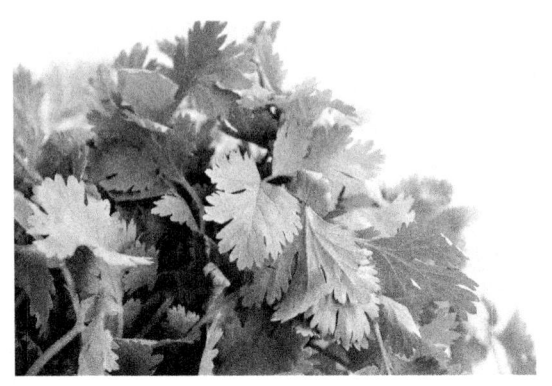

Coriander

Coriander (or Cilantro as it is also commonly known), is often used in Thai and Vietnamese cuisine. It has a strong taste and can take a bit of getting used to if you are not accustomed to its flavour.

Coriander is a herb that I've only added as one of my regulars in the past few years. It has many health-giving benefits, but one that stands out is its ability to **remove heavy metals from the body.**

Coriander works as a natural chelation treatment, removing heavy metals such as lead, aluminium and mercury from the body efficiently and quickly. This is great news for those of us with amalgam fillings as well as anyone who's health is being affected by heavy metal poisoning.

If you don't like the taste of coriander, using cilantro essential oil in a capsule is an alternative way to make use of this herb.

See resources at the end of this book.

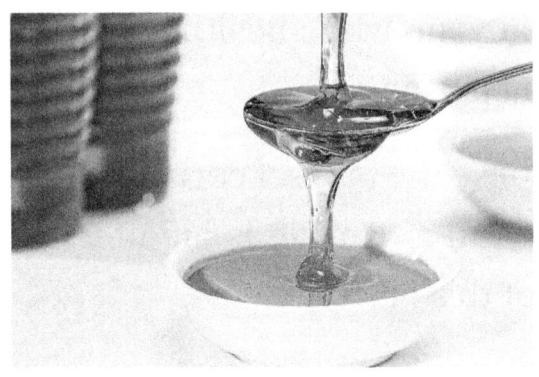

Honey

Honey has been used as a food and a medicine throughout history. Honey is great for colds and flu, as well as sore, inflamed throats.

In recent years the healing properties of honey have become more mainstream, as it has been realized that it is very effective in treating stubborn, resistant leg ulcers as well as other antibiotic resistant bacterial infections such as Golden Staph. Some types of honey are more efficient than others depending on the flora the honey is made from, but all have health giving properties.

Make sure you buy raw unpasteurised honey.

Most brands of honey found in the supermarket are pasteurised. This means they've been heated to a high temperature, killing the beneficial enzymes that raw honey naturally contains, but they generally are not labelled as such.

Some supermarket brands are also apparently cut with sugar or even high fructose corn syrup to make them more profitable. These are NOT the best value for your money!

The best option is always to buy either organic honey or local honey from a market, or even better, buy directly from the beekeeper where it is straight from the hive to the jar. This ensures that you get all the health-giving enzymes and other goodness contained in natural raw honey (these enzymes are killed during the pasteurisation process). If you're buying from a market stall or a beekeeper and you're in doubt, ask if it's raw - that way you'll know for sure.

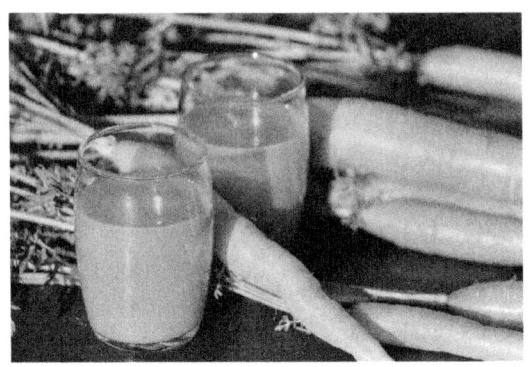

Juicing

Juicing fruits, herbs, and vegetables will give your health an amazing boost - guaranteed. Do it often and make it a habit.

Be careful not to use too much fruit as it can be too much concentrated sugars, although sometimes more fruit is needed for those who are new to juicing and particularly for children. Ideally however, use just a little low sugar fruit such as green apples to make your juice palatable and try to make the bulk of the juice from herbs and vegetables.

I have stages where I juice every morning for breakfast, and a while back I lived on juice only (no solid food) for three months. This is known as 'juice feasting' and is where you consume 3 to 4 litres of juice per day for a period of time. Many people use juice feasting to lose weight and to improve their health. I can tell you that after 3 months on a juice feast, I was 12 kilos down, I felt amazing, and I didn't want to stop. The trickiest part of juice feasting is ending it, and then getting the digestive system working efficiently again - slowly is key! For more info on juice feasting visit http://juicefeasting.com/

Juices are really delicious and they're great for your health. Make sure you include lots of vegetables and herbs in your juices. You can use any variety and combination of vegetables and fruit. Cucumbers are one of my favourites when combined with some carrot, celery and apple. The cucumber juice is refreshing and very cleansing!

Find out which vegetables or herbs might help whatever it is you are working on resolving.

For example, using celery will lower blood your pressure. Add some coriander and you'll be helping to rid your body of heavy metals. Or just add whatever you like the taste of! It's quick and simple, and your body will love you for it.

Fresh juices are almost always used in natural treatments for serious health issues such as cancer, and they can be very effective. But my suggestion is to use them as part of a preventative program to help keep you healthy and to prevent cancers and other diseases. It is much simpler and more efficient to prevent disease than trying to resolve a health problem once it's appeared!

Chapter 16
Recipes & Reminders

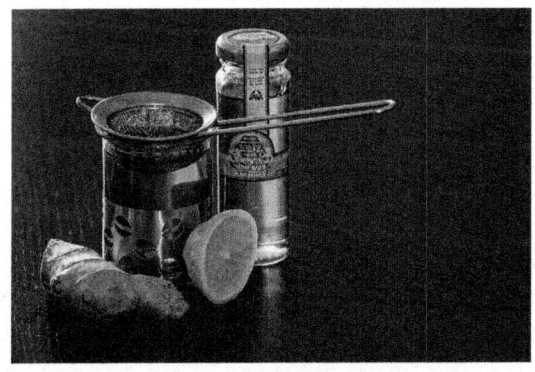

I've added this additional chapter in this later version of this book in response to feedback, and to make it simpler to find the best recipes and main points about remedies that I've included throughout the book. This

section includes the recipes that I personally find the most valuable. I hope you do too.

Slippery Elm

Basic recipe for digestive health

- 1 large teaspoon of slippery elm power
- 1/2 to 1 cup of cold or hot water

Mix well and drink.

Basic Slippery Elm Poultice

- 1/2 to 1 teaspoon slippery elm powder
- Enough water to make a thick paste

Combine well and apply using a sticking plaster or bandage to hold in place. Leave on for 12 to 24 hours and repeat as necessary.

ACV & Slippery Elm Poultice

- 1 teaspoon of slippery elm powder
- 2 or 3 of drops of lavender oil

Enough unpasteurised apple cider vinegar to form a paste

Combine until a thick paste and apply using a sticking plaster or bandage to hold in place. Leave on for 12 to 24 hours. Repeat as necessary.

Garlic

Super simple Guacamole

- 1 clove garlic
- 1 ripe avocado
- Celtic sea salt or Himilayan Salt
- Freshly ground black pepper

Crush the garlic and add to the Avocado. Mash well and season to taste. Enjoy!

Garlic 'Pills'

Crush a clove of garlic slightly then cut into small pieces. Swallow the pieces whole with water as you would a pill.

Note: This works well for some people, but it is probably best taken with food and be aware that garlic may cause indigestion in some people.

Chili

Add chili or cayenne to coffee, teas, and cooking for a bit of health-giving heat.

Aloe Vera

Apply fresh aloe vera gel straight from the leaf to the skin to soothe burns, skin conditions, itching and more.

Make aloe vera juice by blending the gel from one or two leaves with the juice of a lemon and two litres of filtered water. Make sure you blend well. Then pour into glass bottles and refrigerate. This will keep in the fridge for a few days.

Ginger

Ginger Tea

-

- 4 or 5 thin slices of fresh ginger
- 1 cup of water

Add the ginger to an empty cup. Fill with boiling water and then cover with a plate or lid. Allow to steep for about five minutes. Add honey and/or lemon to taste if desired.

Thyme

Thyme Tea

- 1 to 2 teaspoons of fresh thyme leaves
- 1 cup boiling water

Add thyme and boiling water in a cup and cover for 5 minutes. Ginger, Lemon, and Honey can also be added for additional flavour and health benefits.

Lemon

Lemon Water

Add sliced lemon to either filtered tap water or sparkling mineral water. Easy!

Tip: Add stevia to the lemon and sparkling water for a healthy and super quick lemonade.

Fennel

Fennel Seed Tea

- 1 teaspoon fennel seed
- 1 cup boiling water

Add the water to the fennel seed in a cup and cover for 5 minutes. Ginger can also be added to create a tea that is great for calming a windy or upset belly.

Lemon Balm

Lemon Balm Tea

- 2 or 3 sprigs of lemon balm
- Boiling water

Combine in cup and cover for 5 minutes. Add honey if desired. Very useful for calming the body and the mind. Very relaxing!

Apple Cider Vinegar

ACV & Honey Drink

- 1 tablespoon apple cider vinegar (unpasteurised)
- 1 cup hot water

Combine the ACV and honey and enjoy.

Resources: Get Started on Further Research

REMEDIES GENERAL

http://www.earthclinic.com/

Slippery Elm

http://www.umm.edu/altmed/articles/slippery-elm-000274.htm

Baking Soda

http://www.curenaturalicancro.com/en/

http://drsircus.com/medicine/sodium-bicarbonate-baking-soda

http://www.naturalnews.com/027481_prostate_cancer_baking_soda.html

http://www.earthclinic.com/Remedies/baking_soda.html

Apple Cider Vinegar

http://www.earthclinic.com/Remedies/acvinegar.html

Essential Oils

For more information or to buy essential oils that are pure and suitable for internal use visit my website: **Click here for more information**

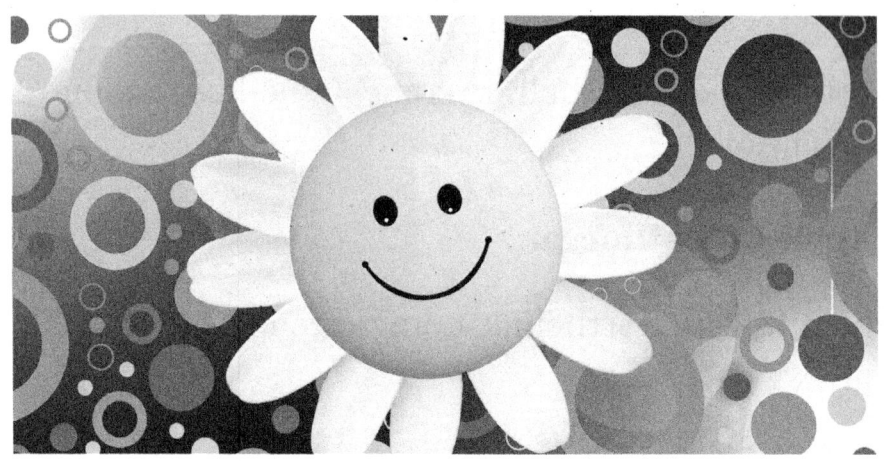

I want to say **Thank You** for downloading this book and for reading and reviewing it on Amazon. I value your feedback and your reviews always help to make future versions and future books better. Thank you so much!

For more books by this author please visit: http://www.amazon.com/Sue-Woledge/e/B0096LO2SU

Printed in Great Britain
by Amazon